Forward

Laughing Venus is dedicated to supporting and enhancing female friendships. **365 Ways to Weasel Your Way Out of Sex: What Every Woman Should Know** is a humorous book that is sure to stimulate conversation and generate a night full of laughs while out with the girls.

365 Ways to Weasel Your Way out of Sex:

What Every Woman Should Know

Marie Chablis & Addie Michel

A LAUGHING VENUS™ BOOK

Published by Laughing Venus™
www.laughingvenus.com

First Printing November, 2008

ISBN 1-4392-1480-8

Acknowledgments

Thanks to our wonderful, loving husbands who, despite the subject matter, supported our vision to create a humorous reference book that enhances our female friendships. Their feedback with respect to content was taken into consideration-but ultimately rejected -and their suggestion to publish this book under pen names was well received and agreed upon.

We treasure the multitude of girlfriends we have in our life and appreciate the fun, unique and unexpected suggestions they provided for the book. Finally, thank you to our awesome graphic arts designer, Kathy Wendt and our other family members who supported us in unique and unspoken ways!

Disclaimer

Girls, it should go without saying, but we still think it's a good idea to remind you . . .please take these ideas in the spirit in which they are intended. These are funny thoughts to generate laughs and good times with your girlfriends.   Please use common sense if you actually desire to put any of these into practice. Just as an example, don't actually bring the bee to bed!

Contents

A Note from the Authors

365 Ways to Weasel Your Way Out of Sex: What Every Woman Should Know was inspired by numerous conversations we had with girlfriends over a glass of wine or a great meal. We were compelled to write this book because we felt most women could identify with and find humor in the subject matter. It is our desire that it will be shared with friends in a lighthearted manner and that laughter will ensue. Enjoy!

First things first.

Let's face it...we all share in the sisterhood of the modern day Venus. Of course, we're goddesses of love and beauty, and of course our man can't resist us. But unlike the Venus of love, we live in the twenty-first century, so in addition to our "love duties," we also need to manage the kid activities, ace the big work presentation, grab the groceries, prepare (sometimes) nutritious gourmet meals, plant the spring pots, and on and on and on. It's pretty clear: with our busy lives, something's got to give.

Any guesses?

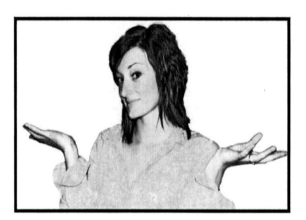

That *something* tends to be at the end of the day, when we're really tired from our crazy schedule.

We can always do that *something* tomorrow.

That *something* starts with an S and falls somewhere down the list of nighttime S priorities, well behind *sleep*.

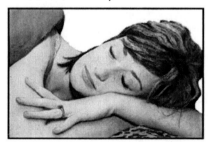

Following the S is an E standing for *every*.

Every time you're drifting off into la la land, you can count on your partner being ready to romp.

Every time you think you've snuck into bed without awakening him, *ping!*

Every woman we know understands what we're talking about.

X, the last letter in this word, stands for *excuse*. That's where this book comes in.

We all love our partners, and maybe to their surprise, we actually do enjoy sex. And yes, we could barely wait to jump into bed when we first met. But as the years went on we became well aware of the fact that our man's sexual appetite was a bit larger than ours, and quite frankly, most nights *we just want to go to sleep!* Do we really need to read another book on how to ignite the spark, rekindle the romance, or find our passion? No! What we *do* need is a simple little book telling women what they really want to know: **How can I get into bed tonight without arousing my partner?**

17

We've all been there...stalled in the bath, read a magazine until we think he's asleep, claimed sheer exhaustion, right? Speaking of exhaustion, you may have exhausted many of your tried and true excuses, and that's where this book can really help. We're here to present fresh, new ideas to eke out one more night of undisturbed relaxation.

Here we go!

Chapter 1

Set the Man Straight

Does your sweetie constantly rely on these "self-recorded" statistics that so-and-so is doing "it" eight times a week, or this guy gets a blowjob every time his wife has her period?

Well...here are a few statistics we've found that you may want to be ready to pull out of your mental bank.

Married couples make love a robust 98 times per year, while single folks are having sex only 49 times a year. *He should consider himself lucky he's married!*

12% of couples in America don't even sleep in the same room. *Again, tell him to consider himself lucky—he could be on the couch!*

57% of people say they have sex at least once per week. *So let him know you may be a bit short, but well within the norm.*

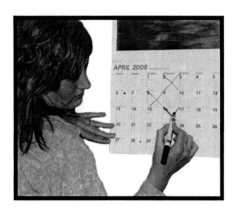

The average couple in their forties has sex 69 times a year (no pun intended!). The average couple in their thirties reportedly does it 86 times a year. The average couple in their twenties does it 112 times a year—*positive proof that one gets wiser with age.*

4% of respondents to a survey claim to have sex daily. *Certainly no one we know.*

People around the world would rather go out with their friends than have sex. More than one-fifth of people chose spending time with their peers rather than having sex with a partner, while another 10% prefer either to play sports or to go shopping. *See, I am normal! Now where was that sale?*

Now that you're armed and dangerous with your own version of sexual reality, it's time to lay the ground rules in your relationship.

Chapter 2
Lay the Ground Rules

It's important to set expectations up front. Defining the ground rules helps your man understand when he *can* and *cannot* initiate sex. Once established, if he can find a time that *is* acceptable to initiate sex, let him go for it. You'll have plenty of outs!

Ground Rules:

Simply tell him, "Honey, there will be no sex..."

1)   in the middle of the night, once I've fallen asleep

2)   once you've fallen asleep

3)   if you roll over and say, "Do you want to fool around?"

4)   if you roll over and say, "Do you want to make love?"

5)   for twelve weeks (at least) after having a baby

27

"Honey, there will be no sex..."

6)   involving an alternate hole

7)   if you're lying in bed naked and waiting for it

8)   if you're drunk

9)   if you fart under the covers

10) without foreplay/romance

"Honey, there will be no sex..."

11)   if you rub up against me like a pervert

12)   if you mention it earlier in the day

13)   if I have my period or am expecting it that night

14)   if the kids are awake

15)   if you piss me off earlier in the evening

"Honey, there will be no sex..."

16)   if I've overeaten and feel bloated.

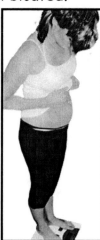

"Honey, there will be no sex…"

17)   if you wake me up early in the morning to have sex

18)   when we have overnight guests

19)   if we're in our parent's house

20)   if the kids have an overnight guest

21)   if the kids are sick

Given the way men tend to operate, these ground rules alone should help you weasel you way out of sex up to 20% of the nights, buying you immediate slumber for **73** nights of the year!

Free Passes

Without a doubt, every woman deserves a minimum of one free pass per month...no questions asked. This buys you *twelve* additional nights of slumber (**FREE PASS** - noted throughout book)

Chapter 3

Set the Tone Early in the Day

There are little "things" that you can do during the day to increase your odds of success at weaseling your way out of sex. An ounce of prevention goes a long way. Here are just a few examples:

22)   Tell your husband that if he does the laundry, makes dinner, cleans the kitchen, gives the kids a bath, reads to each child individually, and puts the kids to bed, you'll have sex. He'll fall asleep!

23)   Mention, as he heads out the door for work, that you've noticed he has some early signs of dementia, i.e. forgetfulness. That night climb into bed and tell him that even though you thoroughly enjoyed your sex last night, twice, and this morning, you now need your sleep. Oh...did he forget?

24)   Power-shop all day and leave the receipts and shopping bags all over the house. Do this on the day you get your credit card bill. This will surely lead to a lecture, argument, and your refusal to have sex on the grounds he doesn't support your passion.

25)   Get up early in the morning to make a pan of gourmet laxative brownies to pack in his lunch for dessert. Be sure to send a couple of extra for a mid afternoon snack.

26)   A good Feng Shui bedroom promotes sensual energy. Create an anti-Feng Shui environment in your bedroom by filling it with your TV, computer, and exercise equipment; close all windows to keep fresh air out; have only bright can lights installed; paint your bedroom a shockingly bright color; place sad and lonely pictures on the wall; push two sides of the bed up against a wall and place bed in direct line of the door; have only one bedside table and keep all doors open at night. It may also help to leave clothes lying all over the floor. He may trip and get too irritated to perform. Admittedly, most men won't care if the room is void of "sensual energy"—so refer to the other ideas in this book if needed!

If you fail to set the tone during the day, you'll be forced to move onto Plan B: Stalling Techniques.

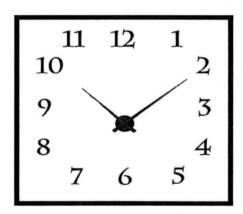

Chapter 4
Stalling Techniques

Stalling techniques are suggested methods to kill time while waiting for your partner to fall asleep. If he wakes up, default to Ground Rule #2.

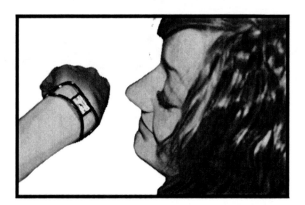

27) Lie with your child to help them "get to sleep"… of course you
       accidentally fall asleep yourself.

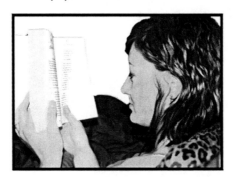

28) Finish your novel.

29) Pull out the old douche kit and enjoy.

30) Color-code the files in your file drawer.

31) Dust the chandelier.

32) Clean up a few e-mails.

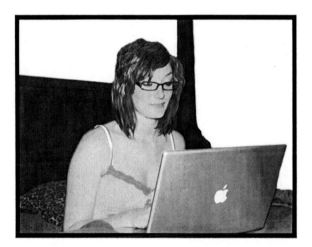

33) Organize your closet.

34) Use Google® to seek out potential vacation spots for spring break.

35) Shop eBay®.

36)   Fold those three loads of laundry that have been lying next to the dryer forever.

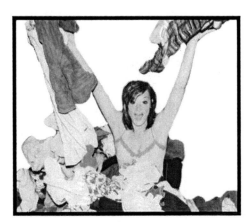

37) Speed-dial a girlfriend on the phone, then talk for an hour.

38) Organize the junk drawer; we all know that will take until morning!

39) Polish the silver—haven't you been meaning to get to that?

40) Organize the recyclables.

41) Have a venti, triple shot, half soy, quarter mocha, part skim latte.

42)   Call your sister.

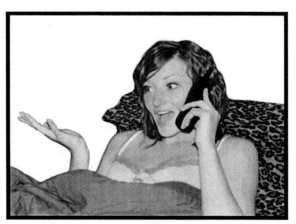

43)   Finish off that bottle of wine.

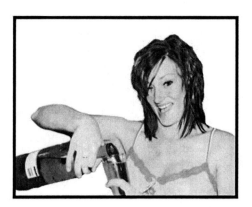

44) Buy him a new video game and have him try it out before bed.

45) Replace the batteries in the smoke detectors.

46) Have a midnight snack.

47) Play "hide and seek" and hide in a really good place. Eventually he'll give up and go to bed.

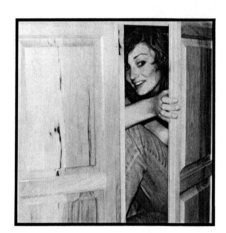

48)   Ask him to run to the grocery store to pick up some feminine pads for you.

49)   Watch your TiVo® shows.

50)   Get everything ready for your "early" business meeting tomorrow: iron clothes, polish shoes, polish jewelry, paint nails…as one thing leads to another, you'll be cleaning out all of the old shoe polish and sorting through your entire jewelry chest.

51) Bring out that large bag of new clothes you've been hiding and insist on trying everything on for him, including every combination that would work from your closet with these new clothes.

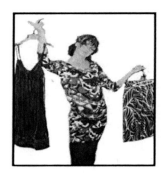

52)   Catch up on a celebrity gossip magazine.

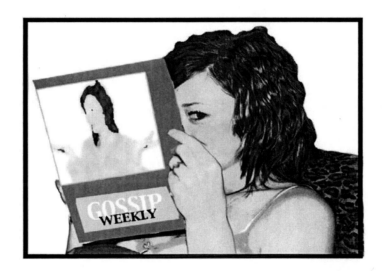

53) Take a long route home from dropping off the babysitter...in fact, consider house hunting.

54) FREE PASS

55) Whiten your teeth.

56) Replace any burnt out light bulbs.

57) Explain that you've been struggling with insomnia and you plan to stay up very late tonight so you will get really tired and can stay asleep.

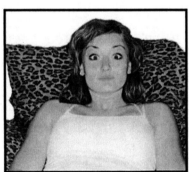

58)   Talk about his ex. Does he still think about her, does he compare you to her, it hurts to think he may, even if he says he doesn't the thought still hurts....

59)   Ask him how many partners he's had and casually mention that you've had more but don't want to talk about it...this could launch into a three-hour conversation.

60)   Tell him you've been waiting all week to see a certain person on Jay Leno tonight and don't want to be distracted.

61)   Do an enema in bed, hop on the toilet, and yell to him that you need to wait until it all drains out.

62)   Pop in a **Do Not Disturb (DND)** bath bomb and relax in the bath for a couple of hours.

63)   Call a girlfriend to discuss your peculiar vaginal discharge.

64)   Tell him he needs to shower first.

65) Text incessantly.

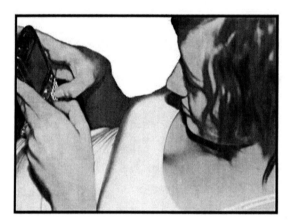

66) Watch a "tear jerker" movie and bawl in bed.

67) Play your new Wii™ exercise game...not in the bedroom, for obvious reasons.

68) Call a girlfriend while in bed to discuss what a "normal" penis size is.

69)   Do the extra hard Sudoku® puzzle in today's paper.

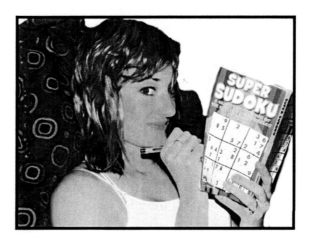

70)   Do a manicure and pedicure and tell him you need to wait for your nails to dry.

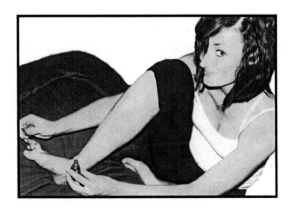

71)   Tell him you need to do 250 Kegel reps to tighten that area for next time.

72)   Tell him you just did a suppository and need to wait until it's absorbed.

73)   Be nostalgic and work on a Rubik's Cube®.

74) Do your nightly meditation and repeat "ohm" quietly at first, then progressively louder, for about two hours. Tell him if he interrupts you, you'll have to start over.

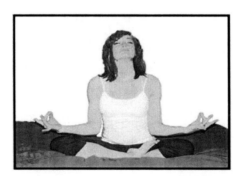

75)   Mention that he ripped you last time with his large manhood and you need a few days to heal.

If stalling techniques aren't producing the results you're looking for, you need to take more drastic measures. Consider the following techniques to physically turn him off so he won't even want to have sex...perhaps ever again!

Chapter 5
Turn-off Tactics

Turn-off tactics are your "nuts" and "screws" (no pun intended) to get out of sex.

Physical Turn-offs

Some physical turn-offs will require a *Turn-off Prop (TOP)*.

76)   Body odor—throw the deodorant out the window.

77)   Come out of the bathroom with toilet paper hanging out of your panties or jammies.

78)   Halitosis—eat roasted garlic right before bed and breathe on him, or let your mouth get very stale and sleep on his chest, gazing up at him with your mouth open, exhaling a sigh of contentment.

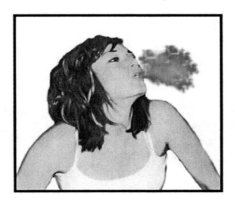

79) Big bushy bush **(TOP #1—a faux piece of fur applied to the pubic area).**

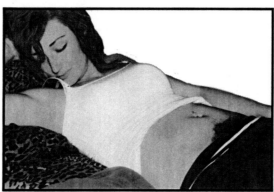

80) Have explosive diarrhea in the master bath before bed **(TOP #2—a laxative or gas-producing dinner).**

81) Wear a pair of Depends™ to bed and say, "Sorry...I'm experiencing incinence" **(TOP #3 – an adult diaper).**

82) Nipple hair **(TOP #4—individual false eyelashes—attach single lashes to nipple or areola to create breast hair).**

83) Nose hair **(TOP #4—attach single lashes to the inside of nose, creating visible nose hair).**

84) Chin hair **(TOP #4—attach multiple lashes to the chin area creating a beard).**

85) Mustache **(TOP #4 - attach single lashes to edge of mouth creating a girl "stache").**

86) Place an extra large dildo, enhanced with hair, on his pillow **(TOP #5 – an extra large dildo).**

87) FREE PASS

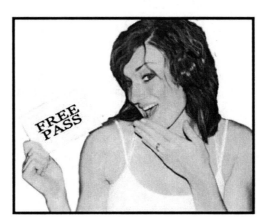

71

88) Leave yeast infection medication on the nightstand **(TOP #6—yeast infection medication)**. FYI.... Yeast infections can last for a month or so.

89) Place bladder infection antibiotics on the nightstand **(TOP #7—an old antibiotic bottle with vitamins inside-he'll never look!)**.

90) Fake a period stain in the **bed (TOP #8—mix red food coloring with corn syrup)**.

91) Wear a pair of large granny underwear to bed **(TOP #9—an old pair of your mother-in-law's underwear).**

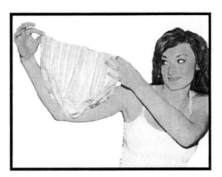

92)   Clip your toenails in bed.

93)   Wear a pair of underwear with a string hanging out of the bottom **(TOP #10—a pair of full bottom underwear with small rope attached signifying a very heavy period!).**

94)   Wear a long, braided pubic hair extension to bed **(TOP #11—a long piece of faux hair attached to your pubic area by microscopic clips).**

95)   Leave an ovulation kit on the nightstand **(TOP #12—a digitized ovulation kit with five sticks laying out, one stick <u>used</u> to show you're serious).**

96) Put a framed picture of the parents/in-laws on the nightstand and mention how much you miss them.

97) Place a Rosie O'Donnell photo on nightstand.

98) Come to bed with hair/food stuck in your teeth.

99) Leave an MD script pad with the words "highly infectious" written on it **(TOP #13—MD script pad)**.

100) Fake an extended case of hiccups.

101) Do an all night mud mask before bed.

102) Fake snoring.

103) Fake farting **(TOP #14—Whoopie Cushion**—place under your buttocks and continue to roll onto it).

104) Get into bed and put on a C-PAP machine for sleep apnea. Your husband will think he's sleeping with an alien.

105) Place hemorrhoid cream on the nightstand **(TOP #15—bottle of Preparation H®)**.

106) Bleach your mustache.

107) Push out some real bad gas.

108) Reverse-tweeze your brow by taking **TOP #4** and filling in the area between your brows to cause a unibrow.

109) Develop a tick.

110) Apply a faux canker sore **(TOP #16—one of your kid's Halloween tattoos that resembles an oozing sore).**

111)   Drop a log in the master bathroom just before bed and forget to flush. ☺

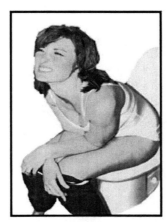

112) Fish oil body smell **(TOP #17—rub contents from a bottle of fish sauce on your inner thighs).**

113) Pretend to squeeze pimples on the inside of your thighs and buttocks in bed.

114) Shave the bush quickly before bed, then place bandages all over the pubic area.

115) Leave a huge maxi pad on the bed.

116) Wear the same panties all week.

117) Pick a booger...and if desperate, eat it.

118) Get into bed with dingleberries (toilet paper balls) hanging from your bush.

119) Eat tons of beans for dinner, creating a distended stomach in addition to gas.

120) FREE PASS

121) Put a raisin in your nose to develop a nose whistle.

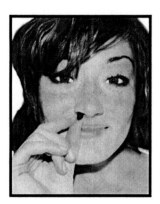

122) Don't shave your arms/legs for a month.

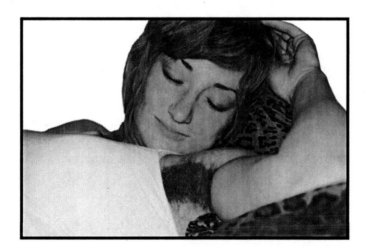

123) Ask him if he'll check to see if your anal warts have shrunk since applying meds, or ask him if he wants you to check his rear for anal warts.

124) Go to bed with a milk mustache.

125) Put a smelly baby diaper on the bed.

126) Eat asparagus for dinner and pee in the master bathroom before bed.

127) Relocate the cat's litter box to under your bed.

128) Dye your entire pubic hair area gray and ask your husband if he thinks you're getting a couple of stray strands of gray hair "down there."

129) Read a book in bed about how to conceive after forty.

130) Offer to massage his genital area and accidently grab the Icy Hot®.

131) Ask him to be careful not to touch your hernia bump.

132) Apply skid marks to your underwear using a dark chocolate bar.

133) Come out of the bathroom "stringing" your egg white ovulation mucus between your fingers.

134) Ask him if he'll insert a suppository for you before bed.

135) Wear men's underwear to bed—though this may be a turn on to some men.

136) Wear an extra large menstrual pad that sticks out of the front and back of your underwear.

137) Wear "old fashion" hair rollers and a robe to bed.

138) Place a wood tick in your pubic hair and ask your husband to pull it out.

<u>Medical Turn-offs:</u>

Keep this book by your bed to be used as a quick reference for signs and symptoms that help you fake an illness with confidence. Illness requires plenty of rest and time to recover. Any energy expended doing an unnecessary act will take away from your body's ability to heal!

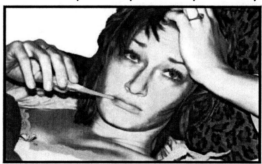

Remember to over-exaggerate and visualize that Oscar®-winning performance! Here are some tid bits of information to help you accomplish your goal.

139) Appendicitis—pain in the middle of your belly.

140) Gall stone—indigestion and pain in the upper right part of your belly.

141) Kidney stone—stabbing pain in the side and back below the ribs that tends to come in waves.

142) Strep throat—throat pain (highly contagious: do not lay facing husband, let alone do the act!).

143) Ringworm—small, red circles or ovals all over your body. These can be made easily with a red pen.

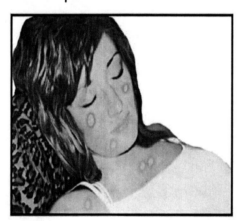

144) Flu—pain in your back, arms and legs, headache and fatigue...how many of us don't have at least one of these symptoms daily anyway?

145) Abscessed tooth—pain in jaw, horrible smelling mouth.

146) Bells palsy—weakness of one side of the face, may become impossible to close one eye (keep one eye open and drop one side of your mouth).

147) Asthma attack—heavy wheezing. Sit down halfway up the steps, take deep breaths, and tell him you need to rest.

148) Chicken pox—small fluid filled blisters on face and trunk. (Give yourself small hickies all over your body put drops of oil on a few and tell him you were exposed).

149) Earache—point to your left ear and tell him you have severe ear pain. If necessary, drip some honey near your earlobe. CAUTION: do not apply honey to any other part of your body!

150) PMS—mood changes, irritability, fluid retention, bloated stomach, tender breasts.

151) Herpes—pain, tenderness or itchy sensation, blisters or open sores.

152) Yeast infection—itching and irritation of the vagina, thick white discharge.

153) Slipped disk—sore neck, intense pain in your back, burning pain down one or both legs.

Mental Turn-offs

If you husband is rip-roarin' and ready to go, mental turn-off techniques may squelch his libido.

154) Make the statement, "I'll lay here, just get it over with."

155) Blurt out the wrong name.

156) Put in a *Dick Does Dan* porno movie to watch together.

157) Talk to your husband in baby talk: "Mommy's going to..."

158) Suggest starting with a *very* large dildo and then having your partner "finish it up." (**TOP #5**).

159) FREE PASS

160) Suggest "talking about your feelings" before sex.

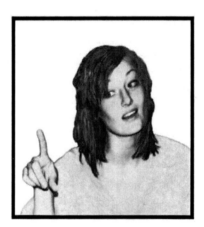

161) Name your body parts after your in-laws.

162) Say, "Let's make a baby."

163) Mention a story you think you heard on the news regarding a new sexually transmitted disease that you can get from toilet seats and that you may have some of the symptoms.

164) Climb into bed with rosary beads and pray.

165) Tell him your IUD fell out today...you can still make love, but you
       may get pregnant.

166) Hand him a bottle of **Dude Lube™** and tell him to take care of it
       himself.

167) Tell him your period is late.

168) Mention that you have a gynecological appointment tomorrow and
       how gross that would be for the doctor.

169) Stick an annoying, repetitive musical toy in the bed that is set off by motion or voice.

170) Slip into a hand-me-down outfit from your mother and tell him that evidently this outfit really turned his father on.

171) Have a talk about money, renovation projects, etc., before sex.

172) Tell your husband you've decided to pick up the guitar and sit in bed practicing and singing, "Blowin' in the Wind" over and over again until you get it perfect. CAUTION: use of the word *blow* in any context is risky.

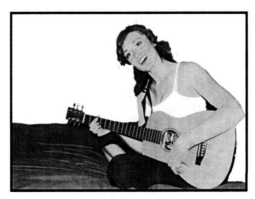

173) Ask him how long he thinks it will take.

174) Let out a few big sighs.

175) Start sobbing about something a friend told you today.

176) Lay there despondent and fake depression.

177) Let him initiate and immediately ask him, "Are you done yet?"

178) Have a talk about differences in parenting styles.

179) Bring up your father/mother-in-law.

180) Sing the *National Anthem* while laying next to him in bed, anything for your country.

181) Send subliminal messages (turn away and curl into fetal position).

182) Comment on the article you just read on large penises and ask if you can measure his.

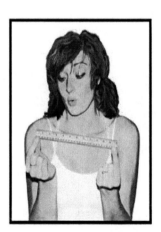

183) Casually say, "I just know I'm ovulating."

184) Eat an entire box of Oreo® cookies while laying next to him (and the crumbs) in bed, and then smile.

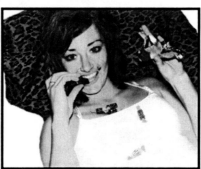

185) Hand him a doctor's prescription stating you must abstain from sex for six weeks due to inactive vaginal muscles **(TOP #13— MD script pad)**.

186) Pinch the "spare tire" around his waist and mention that you're going to hold on for the ride. CAUTION: he may just say okay.

187) Tell him something that irritates him and kills the mood.

188) Ask him if you can squeeze that zit on his back first.

189) Tell him you need to lose just five more pounds and you'll be in the mood.

190) Suggest listening to Barry Manilow music during foreplay.
CAUTION: he may like it...but then you have bigger issues.

191) Mention that you just got notification of a lice breakout in school and your bush feels itchy.

192) Pull out a box of extra-small condoms and say that you special ordered them for him.

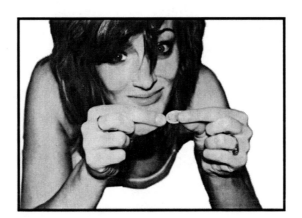

193) Tell him you're still trying to figure out what that inchworm you dug up today in the garden reminds you of.

194) Lay a brochure on the bed that talks about penile enlargement procedures.

195) Tell him you'd rather work off the one or two calories you'd expend tomorrow.

196) Mention how much he reminds you of his father.

197) Get your child's recorder instrument and tell your husband you want him to listen to you practice playing "Bridge Over Troubled Water" until you get it perfect for the kindergarten graduation ceremony. Explain that you need to do this in bed once the kids have gone to sleep, because you want it to be a surprise for little "Tommy."

198) Laugh uncontrollably....and if you can, fart.

199) Mention the doctor appointment you made for him to have an annual rectal exam followed by a colonoscopy.

200) Ask him if he's scheduled his vasectomy yet; if not, no sex.

201) Gag at the mention of a blowjob.

202) Tell him his back hair is a major turn-off and he'll just have to shave before you can get in the mood.

203) Mention that you've noticed he may have the early signs of erectile dysfunction and tell him you've left a message for his physician to call him for an appointment as soon as possible.

204) Ask him if he wants you to be conscious of his premature ejaculation issue tonight.

205) Give him a *Hustler®* magazine and tell him to take care of it himself.

206) Read a transvestite magazine...note the usual caution.

207) Strap on a dildo and tell him you want to try something "different" tonight.

208) Rig a Magic 8 Ball® to always show the words "NO," "NOT TONIGHT," or "DON'T EVEN THINK ABOUT IT."

209) Tell him you want to have a romantic movie night and slip in *Brokeback Mountain*...

210) FREE PASS

211) Give him a blow-up doll to use, but make it a male.

212) If he likes the alternate hole, tell him what's good for the goose....

213) Serve Chinese food for dinner and stuff a fortune cookie with a slip of paper saying, "DO NOT expend any energy in bed tonight, you'll need it all tomorrow. Just wait...you'll see why."

214) If your husband has gray pubic hair, bring a bottle of Grecian® Formula 16® into bed and tell him you really need to spray that area before you can get turned on.

215) Put a plastic mattress protector on the bed.

216) Ask him if you can spray paint his bald spot first.

217) Slap on a pair of **Laughing Venus™** underwear, hop into bed, and point to the graphic stating "Do Not Enter".

Chapter 6
Physical Barriers

Physical barriers are an effective way to buy a free night. Here are some suggestions to get your creative juices going (and not those other juices).

218) Night one: let one of your kids sleep between you, because they need Mama.

219) Night two: let child #2 sleep with between you "to be fair."

220) Night three: let the dog sleep with you so he doesn't feel left out.

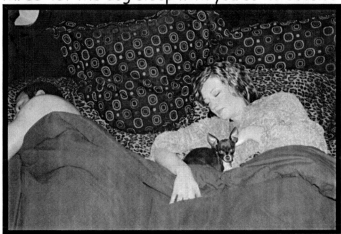

221) Sleep in a full body wetsuit to stretch it out for summer.

222) Go to bed in a sleeping bag.

223) Put a full body pillow in between you and your partner; use Velcro® to attach it to the bed if needed.

224) Place that male blow-up doll between you and your partner in bed.

225) Find an old antique chastity belt, try it on before bed, lock it, and lose the key.

226) Find your husband a job he has to travel for...all the time.

227) Sleep in tight jeans and tell him you need to stretch them out for a fat friend who wants to borrow them tomorrow.

Chapter 7
Vintage Excuses

We've all used these timeless excuses. Sometimes they work and sometimes you meet resistance. Throw them in every once in a while for maximum effect.

228) I have a headache.

229) We just did it last night.

230) I'm beat.

231) I forgot to take my pill.

232) I can feel an aura coming on for a migraine.

233) We're out of condoms.

234) We'll do it tomorrow.

235) I have PMS, so don't even ask.

236) I have lower back pain and may slip a disk.

237) I have a really stiff neck and can barely move.

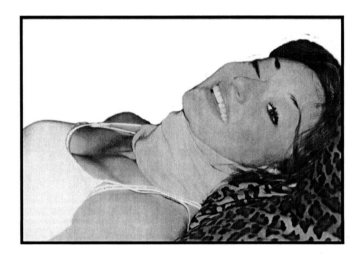

238) I have a stomachache and need to sit on the toilet.

239) I feel bloated.

240) FREE PASS

241) I've decided to be a "born again virgin."

Chapter 8
Special Situation Excuses (SSE)

Take advantage of these golden times in your life to throw out situation related excuses.

General Day-to-Day SSE

242) On Mother's Day—a sex-free night should be part of your gift.

243) On your birthday—you deserve to relax and call the shots.

244) On your child's birthday—giving birth to the kids was exhausting enough. You're entitled to recoup your energy today.

245) Fell off your diet—you already have enough mental stress to deal with.

246) Botched plastic surgery procedure—need time to freak out, then mourn, regroup, call fifteen girlfriends for advice, then go straight to sleep hoping it was just a bad nightmare.

247) Any negative comment from your husband regarding your appearance—automatic "no sex" night.

248) On the day you have to shop for swimsuits—you've seen enough of your body that day.

249) The scale is up five pounds—you're too disgusted with your body to have sex.

Pregnancy Related SSE

Simply tell him...

250) Your water broke or you may have just peed the bed.

251) The baby's head has dropped and he might poke it.

252) You're contracting and can't deal with anything else that's "hard" right now.

253) You both need to get your sleep before the baby comes.

254) You feel nauseous and will puke if you move.

255) You feel like he might crush the baby.

256) FREE PASS

257) If he as much as looks at your breasts, they hurt—so don't even think about coming near you.

258) You just applied hemorrhoid and stretch mark creams.

259) You feel too ugly due to your "mask of pregnancy." Use makeup to enhance your mask so that you resemble a raccoon.

260) You're contracting so hard, it just may snap his penis off.

261) FREE PASS

262) The doctor just told you that you may have sextuplets. ☺
    CAUTION: use of the word *sex* in any context is risky.

263) You just had a prenatal check up and were already poked there once
    today.

264) Sex may cause you to dilate, go into premature labor, be bedridden,
    and then you'd need to hire someone to take care of you, the kids, the
    house, meals, laundry, etc. Is he willing to risk it?

Birth Related SSE

265) Continue to wear your big mesh underpants with a large pad that you got from the hospital after giving birth.

266) Ask him to look at your episiotomy to see if it's healing.

267) Mention you're paranoid of breaking open one of the open wounds on your nipples from breast-feeding.

268) FREE PASS

Menopausal Related SSE

Simply state...

269) I'm dry as dirt down there and may scratch your penis. CAUTION: friction is sometimes what he's after.

270) I'm just laying here in a puddle; if you want to come over and soak with me, feel free.

271) I feel way too bloated and can't have any pressure on my abdomen.

272) I have menopausal related osteoporosis and don't want to risk breaking a bone.

273) My nightgown is wet and I'm not sure if it's hot flashes or incontinence.

274) If you touch me you'll send me into a hot flash.

Holiday Related SSE

Do the following:

New Year's Eve

275) Stall until he's asleep by making a list of all the men you kissed at the strike of midnight over the years.

276) Drink too much and pass out.

277) Drink too much and wet yourself.

Easter

278) Tell him you need to hide the Easter eggs...

279) or fill the Easter baskets...

280) or refuse to entertain the option due to how early you have to get up for Easter sunrise service.

281) FREE PASS

Fourth of July

282) Pretend you can't hear him request sex because you're hearing impaired from the fireworks display.

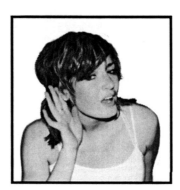

283) Stall until he's asleep by dying your pubic hair red, white, and blue for the holiday. CAUTION: this may turn him on.

Yom Kippur

284) Tell him you're too weak from fasting.

Halloween

285) Tell him you need to sew the Halloween costumes…

286) or bake the pumpkin seeds for the kids snack tomorrow…

287) or you're too tired from trick or treating...

288) or you're too scared...

289) or explain to him that you're too bloated from all of the candy you hand picked out of your kids Halloween buckets and ate.

Labor Day

290) Tell him you couldn't possibly have sex tonight because Labor Day will always remind you of your labor and birth experiences with the kids and how traumatic it was.

<u>Thanksgiving</u>

291) Keep your eyes shut, lay motionless, and complain that the tryptophan in the turkey made you so drowsy you can't even move.

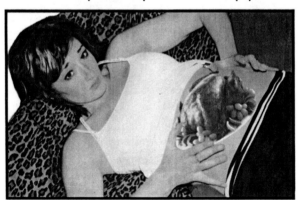

292) Casually mention that you need to get to sleep early and save your energy for the after-Thanksgiving sale tomorrow.

293) Tell him you're bloated from the three pieces of pie (pumpkin, apple and pecan) that you ate for dessert and you need to sleep it off.

Christmas

294) Tell him you need to wrap the Santa gifts...

295) or you need to load the Christmas music on the IPod® ...

296) or you're too stressed out by the sheer amount of money you've spent on gifts...

297) or you're holding out to see how good your Christmas gift is first...

298) or you drank too much eggnog and ate too many Christmas cookies to think about having sex.

299) Since the malls are open until midnight, stay until close.

__Hanukkah__

300) Tell him you are too full from all of the latkes you ate...

301) or too tired from spinning the dreidel all night.

Chapter 9

Emergency Diversion Techniques

Sometimes, one must resort to drastic measures. That's where Emergency Diversion Techniques come into play.

302) Roll out of bed, gently hit your head, cross your eyes, and tell him you're worried about a concussion.

303) Fake Turrets Syndrome—start yelling obscene words out of the blue. CAUTION: don't use the words *fuck* or *screw you!*

304) Pre-record a kid's crying tone on your cell phone and hit this "emergency" button.

305) Cough up a hairball (**TOP #19—hair from your hairbrush),** roll it up into a ball and hold in your palm).

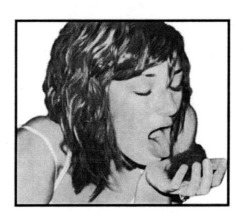

306) Start an argument.

307) Invite your single girlfriend over for a movie night and slumber party. CAUTION: need I spell it out?

308) Pre-record your house security alarm on your cell phone and hit this "emergency" button.

309) Set your pager to go off and pretend you have an urgent work call.

310) Dribble some cherry juice under your nose and on the sheets to
cause a "never ending" nosebleed.

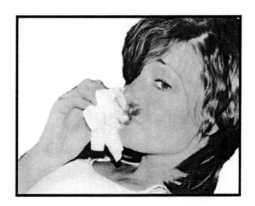

311) Put on a pull up diaper and ask your husband to change you before sex.

312) Pre-record the neighbors fighting on your cell phone and hit this "emergency" button.

313) Pick a poison ivy leaf and rub the essence on the inside of your husband's underwear.

314) Rub nectar on your husband's penis and set a bee free under the covers.

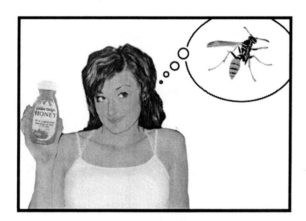

315) Pre-record glass breaking on your cell phone and hit this "emergency" button. Request that he go downstairs to check it out.

316) Have a voodoo doll made of your husband and poke him between the legs before bed.

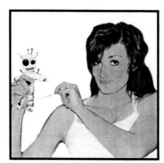

317) Scream at your husband, "YOU'RE NOT GETTING SEX TONIGHT!"

318) Play dead.

Chapter 10
Never Do This

Sometimes preventing arousal is the best tactic. Here are a number of things to keep in mind to avoid igniting the sexual spark.

NEVER...NEVER...NEVER

319) Make any reference to boob, breast, tits, teat, jugs, nipple, boobies, or headlights.

320) Mention penis, cock, dick, shaft, meat, or wank.

321) Say words relating to supple, hard, or stiff.

322) Look succulent when going to bed.

323) Wear sexy negligees, lingerie, thong underwear, fishnet stockings, garter belts, shiny lipstick, push-up bras, g-strings, stiletto heels, or short skirts.

324) Have visible massage gels, lotions, or K-Y® Jelly.

325) Show any nipple or breast tissue (even 1/20 of a millimeter of breast tissue is a turn-on to men).

326) Make any reference to the following sexual toys: vibrating bullet, pocket rocket or g-spot vibrator.

327) Say the words panty or bra.

328) Make any promises with respect to future sex—he'll remember and remind you forever.

329) Allow any part of your body to touch any part of his body, even a toe.

330) Get a Brazilian pubic wax.

331) Reference any fruits including cherry, melon, or peach; and don't eat a banana in the bedroom.

332) Watch a TV show in the bedroom that may have a sex scene.

333) Display titillating magazines or catalogs.

334) Allow any whipped cream into the bedroom.

335) Go to bed naked.

336) Purchase flavored lubricants.

337) Undress in front of him.

338) Talk about your yoga session or say the phrase "downward dog."

339) Allow anything that resembles a pole in the bedroom.

340) Say the words lick, kiss, tongue, or suck.

341) Bend over.

342) In fact, don't even enter the bedroom!

NEVER to Aphrodisiacs

Aphrodisiacs are named after Aphrodite, the Greek goddess of sexual love and beauty. These nasty little encouragers should *not* come in contact with your husband under any circumstances.

343) Oysters—When ordering an appetizer, have the calamari instead. Making a stew? Stick with clam chowder. CAUTION: *clam* is another word you should never mention!

344) Onions—Just use a lot of salt and pecker, I mean pepper, to spice up your burgers.

345) Garlic—If your husband has garlic breath, it's not a good thing—find a quick excuse! Some clinicians have even suggested crushing garlic and rubbing it on the penis as an aphrodisiac. *Don't ever* let your husband rub garlic on his penis!

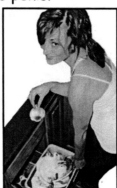

346) Beans—You *know* the added benefit of keeping these away from your husband.

347) Malunggay tea— some sources say that drinking boiled malunggay tea leaves is better than Viagra®!

348) Stay away from the blood or meat of the Philippine cobra which is known to be one of the most venomous and dangerous snakes in the world and is also believed to be a very good aphrodisiac.

349) Rhinoceros horns and penis—especially applicable to women whose husbands have brought back a mounted rhino from an African safari.

350) And...if your husband *is* an African safari kind of guy, beware that certain tiger parts such as the penis, bones, fat, and liver are still being used to make a powerful aphrodisiac soup. If he lands a tiger, *only* the animal's hide is allowed in the house! What's up with animal penis increasing sex drive? Are all male species the same?

351) Betel nuts—areca nuts are seeds of the areca palm tree growing in most tropical countries. These are also known as betel nuts because they are mostly chewed with the betel leaf. This leaf has a peppery taste. Don't ever let your husband shimmy up the areca palm tree while on vacation and pick the nut! If he's a gourmet cook, make sure he's not substituting betel for pepper in his favorite recipes!

352) Never cook with the following herbs or spices: cayenne pepper, cardamom, cinnamon, clove, garlic, mace, nutmeg, parsley, or basil...bland is best!

353) Take out all of the green M&M's®; you can never be too safe!

NEVER Be Home

...as no tactics will work when:

354) He returns from fishing, hunting or any other trips to the wilderness.

355) He returns from a guy trip to Vegas.

356) He gets home after a stag party.

Chapter 11
Times to Suggest Sex

CAUTION—EXPERT LEVEL ONLY—CAUTION

Sometimes, the best defense is a good offense. In this section, we are creating as many moments as possible where you are asking for sex (even begging and pleading). The goal is to ask when you are virtually guaranteed to be turned down, resulting in several occasions to point back to when you are using the tactics provided in the previous sections. "I remember the night when...and you turned me down. I'm not trying to weasel out of sex, our timing is just off. Damn."

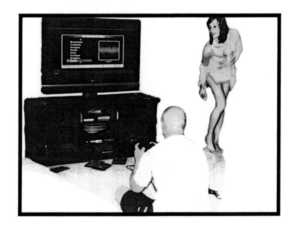

Throw it out there...

357) During the Super Bowl, Masters Tournament, Final Four, Olympics, Stanley Cup, or World Series.

358) After he's up, showered, dressed, heading out the door to work, and running late for his performance review.

359) Right in the middle of an outdoor yard work or garage cleaning project.

360) As he is heading out to play golf.

361) Right after you get back from a long run or workout session and you're dripping wet and smelly.

362) During an intense video game your sweetie is playing.

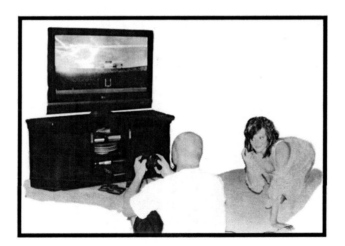

363) When you know guests will be arriving any minute.

364) Right before he heads out to do his Ironman® triathalon.

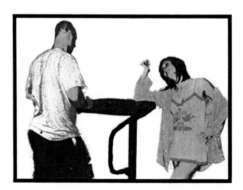

365) Right after he gets home from his vasectomy.

And there you have it...an entire years worth of new, unique and outrageous ways to weasel your way out of sex on those nights that your desire is to sleep instead of romp. And remember, if you do end up giving in...negotiate a little "treat" into the deal!